Beyond the Scale

Understanding and
Overcoming Obesity

by

Helena Mitchell

TABLE OF CONTENT

Introduction

Obesity is a complex and widespread health issue affecting millions of people worldwide. Defined as having a body mass index (BMI) of 30 or higher, obesity increases the risk of various health problems, including heart disease, type 2 diabetes, and cancer.

Despite the well-known risks associated with obesity, many struggle to achieve and maintain a healthy weight.

"Beyond the Scale: Understanding and Overcoming Obesity" is a comprehensive guide that aims to help individuals understand the causes and consequences of obesity and practical strategies for overcoming it.

This book explores the various factors contributing to obesity, including genetic, environmental, and lifestyle factors. It provides evidence-based approaches to weight loss and weight management.

The book is divided into several sections that cover topics such as the importance of nutrition and exercise, behavioral changes, treatment options for obesity, and strategies for long-term weight loss maintenance.

The book also addresses common misconceptions about obesity and offers advice on overcoming setbacks and celebrating successes.

By providing clear and accessible information about obesity, "Beyond the Scale" empowers readers to take control of their health and make positive changes in their lives.

Whether you are struggling with obesity or seeking information to support a loved one, this book offers a valuable resource for understanding and overcoming this complex health issue.

Chapter 1

Understanding Obesity

Obesity is a complex and multifaceted health issue that has become a global epidemic in recent years. According to the World Health Organization (WHO), obesity rates have tripled worldwide since 1975, with an estimated 1.9 billion adults now overweight, of which 650 million are obese.

In this chapter, we will explore the causes and consequences of obesity and misconceptions about the condition.

Causes of Obesity

1. Genetics Research has shown that genetics play a role in obesity. Certain genetic mutations can affect how the body processes and stores fat, making it more difficult to lose weight. However, genetics alone do not cause obesity. Environmental and lifestyle factors also play a significant role.

2. Lifestyle Factors Poor diet, sedentary behavior, and lack of physical activity are key contributors to obesity. Consuming a diet high in calories, sugar, and saturated fats and low in fruits, vegetables, and whole grains, can lead to weight gain. Additionally, sedentary behavior, such as prolonged sitting or inactivity, is linked to obesity.

3. Environmental Factors Environmental factors, such as the built environment, also contribute to obesity.

Factors such as limited access to healthy foods, lack of safe places to be physically active, and social and economic factors can contribute to obesity.

Health Risks Associated with Obesity

Obesity is associated with a range of health risks and conditions, including:

Cardiovascular disease: Obesity increases the risk of developing heart disease, heart attacks, and stroke.

Type 2 diabetes: Obesity is a major risk factor for developing type 2 diabetes.

Cancer: Obesity increases the risk of certain types of cancer, including breast, colorectal, and prostate cancer.

Sleep apnea: Obesity is a major risk factor for sleep apnea, in which breathing is interrupted during sleep.

Common Misconceptions about Obesity

There are several common misconceptions about obesity, including:

1. Obesity is a lack of willpower or personal responsibility that solely causes obesity weight means eating less and exercising more.
2. All individuals who are overweight or obese are unhealthy.
3. Obesity is only a cosmetic issue.

It is important to recognize that these misconceptions are not supported by scientific evidence and can contribute to stigmatization and discrimination against individuals living with obesity.

Overall, obesity is a complex and multifaceted health issue that requires a comprehensive approach to prevention and treatment. The following chapters will discuss evidence-based strategies for overcoming obesity and maintaining a healthy weight.

Chapter 2

Overcoming Obesity through Nutrition

and Diet

A healthy diet is a critical component of weight loss and weight management. In this chapter, we will explore the principles of a healthy diet, the role of nutrition in weight loss, and strategies for incorporating healthy eating habits into your lifestyle.

Principles of a Healthy Diet

A balanced healthy diet provides all the essential nutrients your body needs to function optimally. A balanced diet typically includes the following:

Whole grains: Whole grains are an important source of fiber and nutrients and can help you feel full and satisfied.

Fruits and vegetables: Fruits and vegetables are rich in vitamins, minerals, and fiber and can help reduce the risk of several chronic diseases.

Lean protein: Lean protein sources, such as chicken, fish, and tofu, can help build and maintain muscle mass and keep you feeling full.

Healthy fats: Healthy fats, such as those found in nuts, seeds, and olive oil, can help reduce inflammation and improve heart health.

Strategies for Weight Loss

In addition to following a healthy diet, several strategies can help with weight loss:

Portion control: Pay attention to how much food you eat, and try to eat smaller, more frequent meals throughout the day.

Meal planning: Planning and preparing your meals ahead of time can help you make healthier choices and avoid temptation.

Mindful eating: Practicing mindful eating, or paying attention to the taste, texture, and sensation of each bite, can help you enjoy your food more and avoid overeating.

Tracking your food intake: Keeping track of what you eat and how much you eat can help you identify patterns and adjust as needed.

Coping with Setbacks

Weight loss is not always linear; plateaus are a natural part of the journey. It is important to have strategies for setbacks and avoid feelings of frustration. Some strategies include:

Seeking support: Surrounding yourself with a supportive network of family, friends, or a weight loss support group can help you stay motivated and accountable.

Focusing on progress, not perfection: Instead of fixating on the number on the scale, focus on the progress you are making towards your goals.

Celebrating successes: Celebrate your accomplishments, whether losing a few pounds or making healthier daily choices.

Overall, incorporating this habits into your lifestyle is a key component of weight loss and weight man. By following the principles of a healthy diet and incorporating strategies for weight loss and coping with setbacks, you can achieve and maintain a healthy weight.

Chapter 3

Overcoming Obesity through Physical Activity

Physical activity is a crucial component of weight loss and weight management. This chapter will explore the benefits of physical activity, the types of exercise most effective for weight loss, and strategies for incorporating physical activity into your lifestyle.

Benefits of Physical Activity

Physical activity provides a wide range of benefits for overall health and well-being, including:

Weight loss: Regular physical activity can help burn calories and facilitate weight loss.

Improved cardiovascular health: Physical activity can help improve heart health and reduce the risk of cardiovascular disease.

Increased muscle mass and strength: Resistance training and other forms of exercise can help build and maintain muscle mass and strength.

Improved mental health: Physical activity can help reduce stress, anxiety, and depression and improve mood and overall mental health.

Types of Exercise for Weight Loss

While any form of physical activity is beneficial, certain types of exercise may be more effective for weight loss. These include:

Aerobic exercise: Aerobic exercises, such as running, cycling, or swimming, can help burn calories and facilitate weight loss.

Resistance training: Resistance training, such as weight lifting or bodyweight exercises, can help build muscle mass and increase metabolism, making it easier to burn calories.

High-intensity interval training (HIIT): HIIT involves short bursts of intense exercise followed by periods of rest or lower-intensity exercise and is effective for weight loss.

Strategies for Incorporating Physical Activity

Incorporating physical activity into your lifestyle can be challenging, but several strategies can help:

Start small: Begin by incorporating small amounts of physical activity into your day, such as taking short walks or doing simple exercises at home.

Set achievable goals: Set realistic and achievable goals for your progress towards those goals.

Find activities you enjoy: Choose activities that you enjoy, whether it be dancing, hiking, or playing a sport, to make physical activity more enjoyable and sustainable.

Make physical activity a part of your routine: Schedule physical activity into your daily routine, whether by going to the gym, taking a fitness class, or going for a walk during your lunch break.

Coping with Setbacks

As with diet, setbacks are a natural part of incorporating physical activity into your lifestyle. Some strategies for coping with setbacks include:

Seeking support: Enlist the help of a friend, family member, or personal trainer to provide encouragement and support.

Focusing on progress, not perfection: Celebrate your progress, whether it be by increasing the length of your workouts or trying a new activity.

Reevaluating your goals: If you are not progressing, consider adjusting your exercise routine or setting new, more achievable goals.

Overall, Physical exercise is an important component of weight loss and weight man. By incorporating it you can achieve and maintain a healthy weight being regular physical activity into your lifestyle and using strategies to cope with setbacks, you can

Chapter 4

Overcoming Obesity through Nutrition

Nutrition plays a critical role in managing and overcoming obesity. This chapter will discuss the importance of a healthy diet, strategies for making healthy food choices, and tips for maintaining a healthy diet over the long term.

Understanding the Importance of a Healthy Diet

A healthy diet is essential for maintaining a healthy weight and preventing chronic diseases such as type 2 diabetes, heart disease, and certain cancers. A healthy diet should include the following:

Various fruits and vegetables: These foods provide essential vitamins, minerals, and fiber while also being low in calories.

Whole grains: Whole grains provide important nutrients and fiber while helping regulate blood sugar levels.

Lean proteins: Lean proteins, such as chicken, fish, and legumes, provide important nutrients while low in saturated fat.

Healthy fats: Healthy fats, such as those found in nuts, seeds, and avocados, provide important nutrients and help reduce inflammation.

Strategies for Making Healthy Food Choices

Making healthy food choices can be challenging, but several strategies can help:

Planning: Plan your meals and snacks ahead of time to ensure that you have healthy options available.

Reading labels: Read nutrition labels to understand your foods' ingredients and nutritional content.

Eating mindfully: Pay attention to your body's hunger and fullness cues, and avoid distractions while eating.

Limiting processed foods: Processed foods are often high in calories, sodium, and unhealthy fats, so it's important to limit your intake.

Tips for Maintaining a Healthy Diet

Maintaining a healthy diet over the long term can be challenging, but several tips can help:

Avoid strict diets: Strict diets are often unsustainable and can lead to feelings of deprivation and binge eating.

Find healthy alternatives: Instead of depriving yourself of your favorite foods, find healthier alternatives that you enjoy.

Practice moderation: You don't have to avoid unhealthy foods completely, but practicing moderation and limiting your intake is important.

Seek support: Enlist the help of a registered dietitian or nutritionist to provide guidance and support as you work towards a healthier diet.

Coping with Setbacks

Setbacks are a natural part of the process of improving your diet, but several strategies can help:

Practice self-compassion: Be kind to yourself and recognize that setbacks are a normal part of the process.

Reframe your thinking: Instead of focusing on the setback, focus on the progress you have made and the steps you can take to get back on track.

Revisit your goals: If you need help meeting them, consider revisiting them and making more achievable adjustments.

By understanding the importance of a healthy diet, making healthy food choices, and using strategies to maintain a healthy diet over the long term, you can overcome obesity and achieve a healthier, happier life.

Chapter 5

Overcoming Obesity through Physical Activity

Physical activity is an important component of a healthy lifestyle and can play a key role in overcoming obesity. This chapter will explore the benefits of physical activity, different types of exercise, and strategies for incorporating physical activity into your daily routine.

A. Understanding the Benefits of Physical Activity Regular physical activity can provide numerous benefits, including:

Weight loss: Regular physical activity can help you burn calories and lose weight.

Improved cardiovascular health: Physical activity can help lower your risk of heart disease and stroke by improving your blood pressure and cholesterol levels.

Increased muscle strength and endurance: Regular exercise can help improve your muscle strength and endurance, making everyday activities easier.

Reduced stress and anxiety: Physical activity can help reduce stress and anxiety and improve mood.

Types of Exercise

There are many different types of exercise, each with its benefits. Some of the most common types of exercise include:

Cardiovascular exercise: Cardiovascular exercises, such as running, cycling, or swimming, can improve your cardiovascular health and burn calories.

Strength training: strength training, such as weightlifting or resistance band exercises, can help build muscle and increase metabolism.

Flexibility and balance exercises: Flexibility and balance exercises, such as yoga or tai chi, can help improve your range of motion and reduce your risk of falls.

Strategies for Incorporating Physical Activity into Your Routine

Incorporating physical activity into your daily routine can be challenging, but several strategies can help:

Start small: Begin with short physical activities, such as a 10-minute walk, and gradually increase your activity level.

Find activities you enjoy: Choose activities to make exercise more enjoyable and sustainable.

Set specific goals for your physical activity and track your progress to stay motivated.

Make it social: Join a fitness class or exercise with a friend to make physical activity more enjoyable and hold yourself accountable.

Coping with Setbacks

Setbacks are a natural part of the process of increasing your physical activity. Still, several strategies can help:

Practice self-compassion: Be kind to yourself and recognize that setbacks are a normal part of the process.

Reframe your thinking: Instead of focusing on the setback, focus on the progress you have made and the steps you can take to get back on track.

Adjust your goals: If you need help meeting them, consider revisiting them and making more achievable adjustments.

Incorporating physical activity into your daily routine can improve your health, help you lose weight, and help you overcome obesity. With the right mindset and strategies, physical activity can be enjoyable and sustainable, leading to a healthier life.

Chapter 6

Nutrition and Obesity

Nutrition is a key factor in the development and management of obesity. In this chapter, we will explore the role of nutrition in obesity, the components of a healthy diet, and strategies for improving your eating habits.

The Role of Nutrition in Obesity

Obesity is often caused by consuming more calories than your body needs, leading to excess calories stored as fat. While physical activity plays a role in burning calories, nutrition is the primary factor in managing obesity.

Components of a Healthy Diet

A healthy diet should balance macro-nutrients (carbohydrates, protein, and fat) and micro-nutrients (vitamins and minerals). Some key components of a healthy diet include:

Whole, unprocessed foods: Choose whole, unprocessed foods whenever possible, such as fruits, vegetables, whole grains, and lean protein sources.

Adequate protein intake: Protein is important for building and maintaining muscle mass, which can help improve metabolism and aid in weight loss.

Healthy fats: Include healthy fats in your diet, such as those found in nuts, seeds, avocados, and fatty fish.

Little sugar and refined carbohydrates: Limit your intake of sugar and refined carbohydrates, such as white bread and pasta, which can cause spikes in blood sugar and contribute to weight gain.

Strategies for Improving Your Eating Habits

Improving your eating habits can be challenging, but several strategies can help:

Planning: Plan your meals and snacks to ensure healthy options are available.

Practice mindful eating: Pay attention to your hunger and fullness cues and eat slowly and without distraction.

Practice portion control: Use smaller plates and measure your portions to help control your calorie intake.

Limit processed foods: Limit your intake of processed foods, often high in calories and low in nutrients.

Coping with Setbacks

Setbacks are a natural part of the process of improving your eating habits. Still, several strategies can help:

Practice self-compassion: Be kind to yourself and recognize that setbacks are a normal part of the process.

Reframe your thinking: Instead of focusing on the setback, focus on the progress you have made and the steps you can take to get back on track.

Seek support: Contact friends, family, or a healthcare professional for support and guidance.

Incorporating healthy eating habits into your daily routine can improve your nutrition, manage your weight, and overcome obesity. Healthy eating can be enjoyable and sustainable with the right mindset and strategies, leading to a healthier, happier life.

Conclusion

In conclusion, obesity is a complex and multifaceted condition requiring a comprehensive management and prevention approach. By understanding the factors contributing to obesity, including genetics, environment, and behavior, we can develop effective strategies for prevention and treatment.

Physical activity, behavior modification, medical interventions, and nutrition are crucial in managing obesity. Individuals can achieve lasting weight loss and improve their overall health and well-being by making lifestyle changes and adopting healthy habits.

While overcoming obesity may be challenging, it is important to remember that small changes can make a big difference. Individuals can achieve their weight loss goals and improve their quality of life by taking small steps each day towards a healthier lifestyle.